COLOSTOMY RECOVERY COOKBOOK

Comprehensive Guide Unlocking The Secrets of nutrition after Surgery Success, Nourishing Meal Plans, Recipes And Practical Tips For Optimal Health And Wellness)

DR. ALLAN FREDA

Contents

Welcome to the Colostomy Recovery Cookbook, a thorough manual for handling the post-surgery process with assurance and comfort.

This cookbook is thoughtfully designed to help people who have had colostomy surgery. It offers insightful commentary, useful advice, and delectable dishes that are geared toward fostering healing and overall well-being.

My goal is to arm you with the information and tools you need to face this new chapter with resiliency and vigor since we recognize the difficulties that come with transitioning to life following surgery. This cookbook is meant to be a reliable guide, providing support and motivation at every turn, whether you are starting your recovery path or helping a loved one through theirs. Together, let's set out on this path to a better and healthier tomorrow.

Concerning This Cookbook

The Colostomy Recovery Cookbook is a comprehensive guide to health and recovery, not simply a list of dishes. This cookbook was created by specialists in the domains of holistic health, surgery, and nutrition to cater to the particular requirements and difficulties encountered by those recuperating from colostomy surgery.

Every dish and suggestion is thoughtfully chosen to assist the body's healing process while indulging the senses, with an emphasis on long-term well-being, healing, and sustenance. Every meal, which ranges from colorful salads and filling snacks to substantial stews and warm soups, is carefully prepared to supply vital nutrients, facilitate digestion, and increase vitality.

These pages are full of inspiration, whether you're seeking for quick and simple meals for hectic days or decadent treats for special occasions.

This cookbook offers mouthwatering dishes together with professional guidance on diet, lifestyle modifications, and coping mechanisms to support you while you heal. You may welcome this new chapter with vigor and confidence if you have the correct resources and assistance.

Comprehending Colostomy Healing

The life-altering technique known as colostomy surgery entails rerouting the colon via an abdominal hole called a stoma. This type of surgery is usually done to treat diverticulitis, inflammatory bowel disease, and colorectal cancer, among other illnesses. Although colostomy surgery can provide symptom alleviation and enhance overall quality of life, there is a period of adjustment and recuperation involved. It is imperative to comprehend both the physiological and psychological facets of colostomy recuperation to manage this process with fortitude and elegance.

Physically speaking, recuperating following colostomy surgery entails giving the body enough time to mend from the incisions made during the procedure and adjust to the altered bowel function. As the body gets used to its new digestive mechanism, it's normal to feel uncomfortable, and tired, and have changes in bowel habits during the first post-operative time.

To promote the healing process and avoid problems, it's critical to adhere to your healthcare provider's recommendations for wound care, pain management, and dietary modifications.

Emotionally, living with a colostomy can be difficult and can cause emotions of worry, uncertainty, and anxiety. Many people struggle with issues related to social acceptability, self-worth, and body image as they learn to live with a stoma. During this period, getting help from loved ones, support groups, and medical experts may be extremely helpful.

They can offer comfort, motivation, and useful guidance on how to handle the mental and physical elements of colostomy recovery.

Advice for Successful Recoveries

Following colostomy surgery, recovery calls for persistence, proactive self-care, and patience. Even if the road may have its ups and downs, the following advice and techniques will assist ensure a speedy and full recovery:

1. Observe the advice of your healthcare provider: Your medical team will give you detailed instructions on how to take care of yourself after surgery, including advice on how to manage wounds, how active you should be, and what to eat. To promote the healing process and reduce the possibility of problems, it is imperative that you carefully adhere to the following guidelines.

2. Drink plenty of water: Staying well hydrated is crucial for general health and recovery, particularly following surgery.

To help with digestion and to keep hydrated, make it a point to sip lots of water throughout the day.

3. Consume a balanced diet: A healthy diet is essential for the recuperation process following surgery. To supply vital nutrients and aid in healing, concentrate on eating a balanced diet full of fruits, vegetables, lean meats, and whole grains.

4. Introduce fiber gradually: To minimize discomfort or digestive problems following surgery, it's crucial to introduce fiber gradually. Fiber is essential for supporting a healthy digestive system and preventing constipation. Beginning with meals that are readily digested, progressively add items high in fiber to your diet as you feel comfortable doing so.

5. Listen to your body: Take note of the cues it sends you, and modify your exercise and dietary habits appropriately. If particular meals or activities make you uncomfortable or aggravate

your symptoms, change your strategy and see your doctor as required.

6. Take good care of your stoma: Keeping your skin healthy and avoiding infections needs proper stoma care. Adhere to the suggested stoma care regimen, which includes routine cleaning, fitting the appliance correctly, and keeping an eye out for any indications of infection or discomfort.

7. Remain active: During the healing process, a little exercise can assist in increasing circulation, lessen inflammation, and enhance general well-being. Take care of your body by doing things like walking, yoga, or swimming that make you feel good.

8. Seek assistance: Throughout your healing process, don't be afraid to ask for help from loved ones, support groups, or medical experts. Talking to others who understand your struggles, worries, and accomplishments may be a great way to get support and direction.

You may assist your body's healing process and face the difficulties of colostomy recovery with confidence and resiliency by implementing these strategies into your everyday routine. As you welcome a new chapter of health and well-being, never forget to appreciate each milestone along the road and to have patience with yourself.

Disclaimer

The information in this book is for informational purposes only and should not replace professional medical advice, diagnosis, or treatment. Always consult your physician or a qualified health provider regarding any medical concerns. Do not disregard professional medical advice or delay seeking it based on information in this book.

The author does not endorse or have affiliations with any mentioned entities. References are for informational purposes only.

Consult your healthcare provider before making dietary or lifestyle changes, especially during recovery from surgery, as individual needs vary.

Results may vary, and the information provided is not guaranteed to produce specific outcomes.

By reading this book, you acknowledge and agree to consult your healthcare provider before implementing any information herein.

For further guidance, consult your healthcare provider or reputable medical websites for reliable information on surgery recovery diets.

CHAPTER 1
IMPORTANT NUTRITION FOR THE RECOVERY OF COLOSTOMY

A person's life may be drastically altered by colostomy surgery, requiring modifications to several areas, including eating patterns. To help with healing, manage symptoms, and enhance general well-being, a proper diet is essential throughout the post-colostomy recovery period. This section explores the fundamentals of nutrition that are unique to those undergoing colostomy rehabilitation.

1.1 The Value of a Well-Balanced Diet

For those recovering from colostomies, a balanced diet is essential since it promotes the body's natural healing process and lowers the risk of problems. Essential nutrients include vitamins, minerals, protein, carbs, and fats are found in a well-rounded diet and are necessary for immune system function, tissue repair, and general health. Sufficient nourishment guarantees appropriate hydration, a crucial element in averting dehydration, a prevalent apprehension following surgery. Furthermore, maintaining the consistency of stoma output, controlling bowel movements, and lowering the chance of digestive pain can all be facilitated by a balanced diet.

1.2 Nutritional Guidelines for Patients with Colostomy

Patients with colostomies should follow dietary guidelines that emphasize eating a wide range of nutrient-dense meals while being aware of possible triggers that might impair stoma function or worsen digestive problems. Emphasizing dietary items high in fiber, such as fruits, vegetables, whole grains, and legumes, can aid in controlling bowel movements and averting diarrhea or constipation. However, since some people may first feel gas or bloating, it's important to add fiber gradually and check its tolerance.

Lean meats, chicken, fish, eggs, dairy, tofu, and nuts are among the many foods high in protein that are essential for maintaining and repairing muscle, especially throughout the healing stage. Consuming enough protein can promote muscular growth and wound healing, helping the body rebuild strength and vitality.

Micronutrients, such as vitamins and minerals, are just as important to general health and the healing process as macronutrients. A varied intake of vital vitamins and minerals is ensured by including a range of vibrant fruits and vegetables, which support antioxidant protection, tissue regeneration, and immune system function.

For colostomy patients to maintain good stoma function and avoid issues like electrolyte imbalances and dehydration, they must drink enough water. It's important to stay hydrated throughout the day, especially in warmer regions and when engaging in physical activity. Water is the best option for this.

1.3 Foods Not to Eat While Recovering

To decrease discomfort from their stoma and related problems, colostomy patients may need to limit or avoid specific foods and beverages while adhering to a balanced diet throughout the healing phase. Among them are:

• High-fiber meals: Certain high-fiber diets have the potential to increase stool size and frequency, which might make it more difficult to control the consistency of stoma output. Although fiber is necessary for a healthy digestive system, it's best to gradually introduce high-fiber diets and keep an eye on how they affect stoma function.

• Foods that cause gas: A few foods, including beans, broccoli, cabbage, onions, and carbonated drinks, can cause an excessive amount of gas, which can cause bloating, pain, and increased stoma output. Reducing or eliminating certain foods might aid in discomfort relief and improve comfort in the digestive system.

• Spicy or highly seasoned meals: Strong spices and spicy foods can aggravate digestive system irritation and symptoms like diarrhea or pain in the abdomen. It is best to stay away from very hot or highly seasoned foods, particularly in the early stages of recuperation.

• Odor-causing foods: A few meals, including onions, garlic, certain spices, and seafood with a strong flavor, can make stoma output smell bad. Although odor-control treatments are available, consuming fewer of these meals can help minimize odor-related issues.

1.4 Advice for Meal Planning

Colostomy patients must plan their meals well to meet their nutritional requirements and accommodate any dietary preferences or restrictions.

The following meal planning advice is designed to promote the best possible recovery:

• Emphasize variety: To guarantee adequate nutrient intake and avoid dietary monotony, include a varied range of foods from all food groups. Try varying the flavors, textures, and cooking techniques to enhance the pleasure and contentment of your meals.

• Portion control: Be mindful of serving sizes to avoid pain or overindulgence, especially if your digestive system is still getting used to the new normal after surgery. Large meals might be more difficult to handle than smaller, more frequent meals spread throughout the day.

• Planning ahead: Making meals and snacks in advance can help you save time and energy and maintain a healthy diet, especially on hectic days or when you're tired.

Making meals in bulk and freezing portions will help to guarantee easy access to home-cooked meals.

• Carefully read food labels before consuming packaged or processed foods to find any potential allergens, additives, or ingredients that might make digestive symptoms worse. Whenever possible, choose products with the fewest possible additives and preservatives.

• Seek expert advice: Speaking with a registered dietitian or other healthcare professional who specializes in colostomy care can offer tailored dietary advice and address particular issues or difficulties. They can assist in developing a personalized meal plan that takes into account dietary restrictions, tastes, and requirements.

it is critical for those undergoing colostomy recovery to adopt a mindful and balanced approach to nutrition. Individuals can optimize stoma function, support their healing process, and enhance their quality of life and long-term well-being by following dietary guidelines, avoiding problematic foods, and putting effective meal-planning strategies into practice.

CHAPTER 2

HEALING BREAKFAST RECIPES

Breakfast is frequently considered the most significant meal of the day because it supplies the body with essential nutrients and energy to restart its metabolic processes following a night of sleep.

A healthy breakfast is especially important for those recovering from colostomy surgery because it helps with healing and sets the tone for the day. Here, we explore a range of therapeutic breakfast recipes, with an emphasis on nutrient-dense choices that support recuperation and general well-being.

2.1 Invigorating Smoothies for Breakfast

Smoothies are a great option for people recovering from colostomy surgery because they are a tasty and easy way to get all the nutrients you need in one meal. These vibrant breakfast smoothies contain a variety of fruits, vegetables, protein sources, and healthy fats that are blended to give you a well-rounded nutritional boost to start the day. Leafy greens, berries, Greek yogurt, nut butter, and seeds are a few examples of ingredients that can be added to make a nutrient-dense drink that supports healing and enhances general health. These drinks' smooth texture also makes them easy to digest, which is particularly advantageous for people who have to undergo surgery or have dietary restrictions.

2.2 Oatmeal Varieties Packed with Nutrients

A flexible breakfast option, oatmeal can be tailored to meet dietary requirements and personal preferences. Nutrient-dense oatmeal varieties can give people recovering from colostomy surgery the sustained energy and vital nutrients they need for the best possible healing. While toppings like fresh fruit, nuts, seeds, and spices add taste, texture, and extra nutritional value, whole-grain oats provide a filling base. Because of their high fiber content, oats are especially advantageous for people getting used to living with a colostomy because they facilitate regular bowel movements and aid in digestion. In addition, oatmeal's complex carbohydrates offer a consistent energy source that lasts throughout the morning, preventing fatigue and promoting general well-being.

2.3 Egg Dishes High in Protein

Protein is a vital component of any post-surgery diet because it is necessary for muscle recovery and tissue repair. For those recovering from colostomy surgery, eggs are a great breakfast option because they are a convenient and adaptable source of high-quality protein. Eggs are a great food to eat scrambled, poached, or as part of a savory omelet because they contain the amino acids that the body needs to heal and regenerate. Eggs are also a great source of vitamins and minerals, such as choline, vitamin B12, and vitamin D, all of which are vital for good health. By incorporating protein-rich egg dishes into their morning routine, individuals can support the recovery process and ensure they are meeting their nutritional needs during this critical time.

2.4 Quick and Easy Breakfast Bakes

For those with busy schedules or limited time in the morning, quick and easy breakfast bakes offer a convenient solution that can be prepared in advance and enjoyed throughout the week.

These hearty dishes can be customized to include a variety of ingredients, such as eggs, vegetables, cheese, and lean meats, providing a balanced mix of nutrients to support recovery post-colostomy surgery.

By preparing a batch of breakfast bakes ahead of time, individuals can streamline their morning routine and ensure they have a nutritious meal ready to go, even on hectic days. Additionally, breakfast bakes can be easily customized to suit individual taste preferences and dietary restrictions, making them a versatile option for those navigating the challenges of recovery.

incorporating healing recipes into the breakfast routine is essential for individuals recovering from colostomy surgery.

By choosing nutrient-rich options such as energizing smoothies, nutrient-packed oatmeal, protein-rich egg dishes, and quick and easy breakfast bakes, individuals can support the healing process and promote long-term wellness.

These recipes not only provide essential nutrients for recovery but also offer delicious and satisfying meal options that make the breakfast experience enjoyable and nourishing. With a focus on optimal nutrition and healing ingredients, individuals can take proactive steps toward a successful recovery and improved overall health.

CHAPTER 3
NOURISHING LUNCHES FOR RECOVERY

Recovery from colostomy surgery requires a balanced and nutritious diet that supports healing, energy levels, and overall well-being. Lunchtime presents an opportunity to refuel and nourish the body with nutrient-rich foods that aid in the healing process. In this section, we explore various lunch options tailored to support colostomy recovery, focusing on wholesome soups and broths, colorful salad creations, hearty sandwiches and wraps, and comforting one-pot meals.

3.1 Wholesome Soups and Broths

Soups and broths are excellent options for individuals recovering from colostomy surgery due to their comforting nature and ease of digestion. Incorporating a variety of vegetables, lean proteins, and whole grains can provide essential nutrients necessary for healing and recovery.

Opting for homemade soups allows for greater control over ingredients, ensuring freshness and minimizing the intake of preservatives and sodium. Broths infused with herbs and spices not only add flavor but also offer potential health benefits, such as reducing inflammation and supporting immune function. Whether it's a classic chicken noodle soup or a hearty vegetable broth, incorporating wholesome soups into the post-surgery diet can promote hydration and nourishment, aiding in the healing process.

3.2 Colorful Salad Creations

Salads offer a versatile and refreshing option for lunch, providing a wide array of vitamins, minerals, and fiber essential for optimal recovery post-surgery. Incorporating an assortment of colorful vegetables, leafy greens, and lean proteins can create a nutrient-dense meal that supports healing and promotes gastrointestinal health. Adding sources of healthy fats, such as avocado or nuts, can enhance satiety and provide additional nutrients beneficial for recovery. Additionally, incorporating homemade dressings made from heart-healthy oils and vinegar can further enhance the nutritional value of the salad while avoiding unnecessary additives and preservatives. By embracing vibrant and diverse ingredients, salad creations become not only visually appealing but also a vital component of a post-colostomy surgery diet aimed at promoting long-term wellness.

3.3 Hearty Sandwiches and Wraps

Sandwiches and wraps offer a convenient and satisfying option for individuals in the recovery phase after colostomy surgery. By selecting whole-grain bread or wraps as a base, one can increase fiber intake, promoting digestive health and regularity. Incorporating lean proteins, such as grilled chicken or turkey, provides essential amino acids necessary for tissue repair and muscle maintenance. Adding an assortment of vegetables and spreads, such as hummus or avocado, not only enhances flavor but also contributes essential vitamins, minerals, and antioxidants. Moreover, choosing low-sodium deli meats and minimizing the use of high-fat condiments can help maintain heart health and support overall well-being. Whether enjoyed at home or on the go, hearty sandwiches and wraps offer a satisfying and nourishing lunch option for individuals navigating the recovery journey post-colostomy surgery.

3.4 Comforting One-Pot Meals

One-pot meals offer simplicity and convenience, making them an ideal option for individuals in the recovery phase after colostomy surgery.

By combining various ingredients in a single pot or pan, such as lean proteins, whole grains, and vegetables, one can create a balanced and nutritious meal that supports healing and sustains energy levels throughout the day. Incorporating ingredients rich in vitamins, minerals, and antioxidants can aid in the recovery process and promote overall well-being. Additionally, utilizing herbs and spices to flavor one-pot meals not only enhances taste but also offers potential health benefits, such as reducing inflammation and supporting immune function. Whether it's a comforting bowl of chicken and vegetable stew or a hearty quinoa and black bean skillet, one-pot meals provide nourishment and satisfaction, essential for individuals recovering from colostomy surgery.

CHAPTER 4
SATISFYING DINNERS TO AID RECOVERY

In the journey of post-colostomy surgery recovery, the significance of a well-balanced diet cannot be overstated. Each meal presents an opportunity to replenish the body with essential nutrients, promote healing, and provide comfort. Particularly during dinner, when the day's activities have come to a close, it's crucial to indulge in satisfying yet nourishing dishes. This section delves into various categories of dinner options tailored to aid in recovery, offering a spectrum of flavors and textures to accommodate different preferences and dietary needs.

Flavorful Grilled and Roasted Meats

Grilled and roasted meats stand as quintessential dinner options for those on the path to recovery post-colostomy surgery.

These preparations not only impart robust flavors but also retain the nutritional integrity of the protein sources. Lean cuts of chicken, turkey, beef, and pork are ideal choices as they provide ample protein to support tissue repair and muscle strength without overwhelming the digestive system. Seasoned with herbs, spices, and marinades, these meats offer versatility in flavor profiles, catering to individual tastes and preferences. Incorporating grilled or roasted meats into dinners ensures a satisfying meal that contributes to overall wellness and recovery.

Delicious Fish and Seafood Entrees

For individuals navigating colostomy recovery, incorporating fish and seafood into dinner menus offers a myriad of health benefits. Rich in omega-3 fatty acids, vitamins, and minerals, these aquatic delights promote cardiovascular health, reduce inflammation, and support immune function—all crucial aspects of the recovery process. From salmon and trout to shrimp and scallops, the options are diverse, allowing for creativity in meal preparation. Grilled, baked, or pan-seared, fish and seafood entrees provide a light yet satisfying dinner option that is gentle on the digestive system while delivering essential nutrients for optimal healing.

Vegetable-Forward Main Dishes

Vegetable-forward main dishes serve as an excellent foundation for dinners during colostomy recovery, offering an abundance of vitamins, minerals, and dietary fiber. Incorporating a variety of colorful vegetables such as leafy greens, cruciferous veggies, and root vegetables not only adds vibrancy to the plate but also promotes digestive health and overall well-being.

Whether enjoyed raw in salads, roasted with herbs and spices, or sautéed with garlic and olive oil, vegetables provide essential nutrients while imparting delicious flavors and textures. Coupled with grains or legumes, vegetable-forward main dishes offer a balanced and nourishing dinner option that supports the body's healing processes.

Grain-based bowls and Casseroles

Grain-based bowls and casseroles present a convenient and comforting dinner option for individuals recovering from colostomy surgery.

Incorporating whole grains such as brown rice, quinoa, or barley provides a steady source of complex carbohydrates, fiber, and essential nutrients to fuel the body and promote satiety.

Coupled with an array of vegetables, lean proteins, and flavorful sauces or dressings, grain-based bowls, and casseroles offer a well-rounded meal that is both satisfying and nutritious.

In essence, crafting satisfying dinners to aid in colostomy recovery requires a thoughtful balance of flavors, textures, and nutrients. From flavorful grilled meats to vegetable-forward main dishes, each dinner option plays a crucial role in nourishing the body and promoting healing.

By embracing variety and creativity in meal preparation, individuals can embark on a culinary journey that not only supports their recovery but also enhances their overall well-being in the long run.

CHAPTER 5
HEALING SNACKS AND SIDES

After undergoing colostomy surgery, maintaining a balanced diet becomes crucial for recovery and long-term wellness. This section delves into the realm of healing snacks and sides, offering a variety of nutritious options to support optimal healing and overall health.

Nutritious Snack Ideas

In the realm of post-colostomy recovery, incorporating nutritious snacks into your diet can significantly contribute to your overall well-being. These snacks serve as essential fuel for your body, providing the necessary nutrients to aid in healing and replenishment. Opt for snacks that are rich in protein, fiber, vitamins, and minerals to promote healing and boost energy levels. Nutrient-dense options such as Greek yogurt with fruit, hummus with whole-grain crackers or veggies, nuts and seeds, and hard-boiled eggs can provide a satisfying and nourishing snack between meals. Additionally, incorporating fresh fruits, such as apples or berries, and raw vegetables, like carrots or cucumber slices, can offer a refreshing and hydrating option to keep you feeling satisfied and energized throughout the day.

Creative Veggie and Dip Combinations

Adding a variety of colorful vegetables to your diet post-colostomy surgery not only enhances the nutritional value of your meals but also adds flavor and texture to your culinary experience.

Pairing these veggies with delicious and nutritious dips can elevate your snacking game to a whole new level. Consider creative combinations such as crunchy bell pepper strips with creamy avocado hummus, crisp cucumber rounds with tangy tzatziki sauce, or lightly steamed broccoli florets with zesty lemon-garlic aioli. Experimenting with different veggie and dip pairings allows you to discover new flavors and textures while ensuring that you meet your dietary needs for optimal recovery and long-term wellness.

Homemade Energy Bars and Bites

When it comes to convenient and nourishing snacks for post-colostomy recovery, homemade energy bars, and bites are an excellent choice.

These portable treats are packed with wholesome ingredients that provide a quick and convenient source of energy and nutrition. By making your energy bars and bites at home, you have full control over the ingredients, allowing you to customize them to suit your dietary preferences and needs. Choose ingredients such as rolled oats, nuts, seeds, dried fruits, and nut butter to create delicious and satisfying snacks that are rich in protein, fiber, and essential nutrients. Experiment with different flavor combinations and textures to find the perfect recipe that satisfies your taste buds while supporting your recovery journey.

Incorporating wholesome side dishes into your meals post-colostomy surgery not only adds variety and flavor but also ensures that you receive a well-rounded and balanced diet. These side dishes complement the main courses, providing additional nutrients and dietary fiber to support digestive health and overall wellness.

Opt for nutrient-rich options such as roasted vegetables, quinoa salad, steamed greens, or whole-grain pilaf to accompany your meals. These dishes not only add color and texture to your plate but also contribute essential vitamins, minerals, and antioxidants to promote healing and recovery. Experiment with different ingredients and cooking methods to create delicious and nutritious side dishes that enhance your dining experience while supporting your journey toward long-term wellness.

In summary, healing snacks and sides play a crucial role in post-colostomy recovery, providing essential nutrients, energy, and flavor to support optimal healing and long-term wellness. By incorporating nutritious snack ideas, creative veggie and dip combinations, homemade energy bars and bites, and wholesome side dishes into your diet, you can ensure that you meet your dietary needs while enjoying delicious and satisfying meals throughout your recovery journey. Experiment with different ingredients, flavors, and cooking techniques to discover new favorites and nourish your body for optimal health and well-being.

CHAPTER 6:

DECADENT DESSERTS FOR RECOVERY

Indulgent Fruit-Based Treats:

When recovering from a colostomy surgery, indulging in desserts might seem counterintuitive to maintaining a healthy diet. However, it's essential to find a balance between treating yourself and nourishing your body during this time. Indulgent fruit-based treats offer a delightful way to satisfy your sweet cravings while providing essential vitamins and minerals to support your recovery process. Incorporating fruits like berries, apples, pears, and bananas into your desserts not only adds natural sweetness but also contributes to your overall nutritional intake.

From refreshing fruit salads to vibrant fruit sorbets, there are numerous options to explore that cater to various tastes and preferences.

These treats not only tantalize your taste buds but also promote digestion and provide energy, making them an ideal choice for individuals on the path to recovery.

Guilt-Free Baked Goods:

Baked goods are often associated with comfort and indulgence, but they can also be a part of a healthy post-surgery diet when prepared mindfully.

Guilt-free baked goods focus on using wholesome ingredients and alternative flours to create treats that are lower in refined sugars and carbohydrates, making them suitable for individuals recovering from colostomy surgery. By substituting traditional white flour with whole grain or gluten-free options like almond flour or oat flour, you can enhance the nutritional value of your baked goods while maintaining their delicious taste and texture. Incorporating natural sweeteners such as honey, maple syrup, or mashed bananas reduces the need for added sugars, promoting stable blood sugar levels and supporting overall health.

From nutrient-rich muffins and scones to hearty cookies and cakes, guilt-free baked goods offer a satisfying way to enjoy desserts without compromising your recovery goals.

Comforting Puddings and Custards:

During the recovery period following colostomy surgery, comfort foods play a vital role in providing nourishment and emotional support. Puddings and custards, with their creamy textures and soothing flavors, are ideal choices for individuals seeking comfort without compromising their dietary requirements. By utilizing nutritious ingredients such as low-fat milk, Greek yogurt, and eggs, these desserts offer a good source of protein and calcium, essential nutrients for healing and maintaining muscle strength. Incorporating flavors like vanilla, chocolate, and butterscotch adds a touch of indulgence while ensuring that the desserts remain gentle on the digestive system. Whether enjoyed warm or chilled, puddings and custards provide a comforting treat that satisfies cravings while promoting overall well-being during the recovery process.

Sweet Endings with a Health Twist:

As you navigate the recovery journey post-colostomy surgery, incorporating sweet endings with a health twist can enhance your overall well-being and support long-term wellness goals.

These desserts prioritize nutrient-dense ingredients and innovative techniques to create flavorful treats that contribute to your healing process. By incorporating superfoods such as chia seeds, flaxseeds, and nuts, these desserts offer a boost of essential nutrients, including omega-3 fatty acids and antioxidants, which support inflammation reduction and promote overall health. Additionally, experimenting with alternative sweeteners like stevia or monk fruit extract allows you to enjoy the sweetness without the added calories or impact on blood sugar levels. From nutrient-packed energy balls and granola bars to decadent avocado chocolate mousse, sweet endings with a health twist offer a satisfying way to indulge in desserts while prioritizing your recovery and long-term well-being.

CHAPTER 7

BEVERAGES FOR HYDRATION AND HEALING

After undergoing colostomy surgery, the journey towards recovery involves not only physical healing but also a holistic approach towards wellness, including nutrition. Beverages play a crucial role in hydration, nourishment, and overall well-being during this period. In this section, we will explore various beverage options tailored to aid in colostomy recovery, focusing on rejuvenating smoothies, herbal teas, fruit-infused waters, and nutrient-packed juices and shakes.

Rejuvenating Smoothie Recipes: Smoothies are an excellent way to incorporate essential nutrients, vitamins, and minerals into your diet while ensuring easy digestion and hydration, which are vital during the recovery phase post-colostomy surgery.

These recipes are designed to be gentle on the digestive system yet packed with healing properties. Ingredients such as leafy greens, fruits, yogurt, and healthy fats like avocado or nuts can be blended to create delicious and nourishing smoothies.

For example, a green smoothie made with spinach, banana, avocado, and almond milk provides a powerhouse of nutrients such as potassium, fiber, and healthy fats, aiding in digestion and promoting overall healing. Experimenting with different combinations allows for variety and ensures that you are getting a wide range of essential nutrients to support your recovery journey.

Herbal Teas and Infusions: Herbal teas and infusions offer not only hydration but also therapeutic benefits that can aid in the recovery process after colostomy surgery. Certain herbs possess anti-inflammatory, digestive, and soothing properties, which can alleviate discomfort and promote healing.

Chamomile tea, for instance, is renowned for its calming effects on the digestive system, making it an ideal choice for those experiencing post-surgery discomfort. Peppermint tea is another excellent option known for its ability to relieve bloating and aid in digestion. Additionally, ginger tea can help alleviate nausea, a common side effect of anesthesia or pain medications.

Incorporating these herbal teas into your daily routine can provide comfort and support during the recovery period.

Refreshing Fruit-Infused Waters: Staying hydrated is essential for optimal recovery post-colostomy surgery, and fruit-infused waters offer a refreshing and flavorful way to meet your fluid needs. Infusing water with fruits such as lemon, cucumber, berries, or herbs like mint adds a subtle flavor while providing additional nutrients and antioxidants. These infused waters not only help in maintaining hydration levels but also support detoxification and digestion. Lemon-infused water, for example, aids in digestion and alkalizes the body, while cucumber-infused water is hydrating and refreshing. Experiment with different fruit and herb combinations to find your favorite flavors and stay hydrated throughout your recovery journey.

Nutrient-Packed Juices and Shakes: Juices and shakes can be a convenient and nutrient-dense option for individuals recovering from colostomy surgery, especially for those who may have difficulty consuming solid foods initially.

Freshly pressed juices made from a variety of fruits and vegetables provide essential vitamins, minerals, and antioxidants necessary for healing and recovery. Incorporating ingredients such as carrots, beets, leafy greens, and berries into your juices ensures a diverse range of nutrients to support your body's needs.

Additionally, protein shakes made with ingredients like whey or plant-based protein powder, fruits, and nut butter can help maintain muscle mass and support tissue repair during the recovery process. These nutrient-packed beverages offer a convenient and delicious way to nourish your body and aid in the healing process post-colostomy surgery.

incorporating a variety of beverages into your post-colostomy recovery diet is essential for hydration, nourishment, and overall well-being. Rejuvenating smoothies, herbal teas, fruit-infused waters, and nutrient-packed juices and shakes offer a diverse range of nutrients and therapeutic benefits to support your body's healing process. Experiment with different recipes and ingredients to find what works best for you, and remember to stay hydrated and nourished as you embark on your journey toward optimal recovery and long-term wellness.

CHAPTER 8

CULINARY TIPS AND TECHNIQUES

Cooking is not merely a task; it's an art, especially when it comes to catering to specific dietary needs during the recovery process after colostomy surgery. In this section, we will delve into various culinary tips and techniques tailored to ensure optimal nutrition, enhance flavors, facilitate meal prepping and storage, and introduce helpful kitchen gadgets to ease the cooking process.

Each facet plays a crucial role in the Colostomy Recovery Cookbook, designed to support individuals in their journey toward healing and long-term wellness.

Cooking Methods for Optimal Nutrition

Selecting the right cooking methods can significantly impact the nutritional content of meals, which is paramount for individuals undergoing colostomy recovery. While the primary goal is to retain nutrients, it's also essential to ensure the food is easily digestible and gentle on the digestive system. Steaming is one of the healthiest cooking methods as it preserves the maximum amount of nutrients while keeping the food tender. Boiling is another suitable option, especially for vegetables, as it softens them without adding extra fat. Additionally, baking and roasting can enhance flavors without excessive oil or fat, providing a nutritious and delicious outcome. Grilling is a method to consider for meats and fish, as it allows excess fat to drip away while imparting a smoky taste. By understanding and employing these cooking methods, individuals can optimize their nutritional intake during the colostomy recovery period.

Flavor Enhancing Ingredients

During the recovery phase post-colostomy surgery, maintaining an appetite and enjoying meals is crucial for overall well-being.

Incorporating flavor-enhancing ingredients can elevate the taste of dishes without compromising health.

Herbs and spices such as basil, parsley, turmeric, and ginger not only add depth to dishes but also offer anti-inflammatory and digestive benefits. Citrus fruits like lemon and lime can brighten flavors while providing a refreshing zest.

Additionally, incorporating umami-rich ingredients such as mushrooms, tomatoes, and nutritional yeast can impart a savory depth to meals. Healthy fats from sources like avocados, nuts, and olive oil can add richness and mouthfeel to dishes, enhancing overall satisfaction.

By incorporating these flavor-enhancing ingredients mindfully, individuals can enjoy delicious meals while supporting their recovery journey.

Efficient meal prepping and storage are essential components of managing a post-colostomy surgery diet effectively. Planning meals not only saves time but also ensures that individuals have access to nutritious options readily available.

When meal prepping, it's essential to consider variety, incorporating a mix of lean proteins, complex carbohydrates, and colorful fruits and vegetables. Utilizing portion control containers or meal prep trays can aid in portioning out meals accurately, ensuring a balanced intake.

Proper storage techniques, such as using airtight containers or freezer bags, help maintain the freshness and quality of prepared meals. Labeling containers with the date and contents can streamline meal selection and reduce food waste. Additionally, investing in a vacuum sealer can extend the shelf life of prepared foods, providing convenience without compromising on nutrition. By incorporating these meal-prepping and storage tips, individuals can maintain a nourishing diet throughout their colostomy recovery journey.

Kitchen Gadgets for Easy Cooking

Incorporating the right kitchen gadgets can streamline the cooking process and make meal preparation more accessible, especially during the recovery period following colostomy surgery.

A high-speed blender is a versatile tool that can be used to create smoothies, soups, and purees, providing easily digestible options packed with nutrients. A food processor is invaluable for chopping, slicing, and shredding ingredients, saving time and effort in meal preparation. Investing in a slow cooker or instant pot can simplify cooking, allowing individuals to prepare flavorful meals with minimal hands-on time. For those with limited dexterity or mobility, adaptive kitchen gadgets such as easy-grip utensils and jar openers can make cooking more manageable and enjoyable. Additionally, a digital kitchen scale can aid in portion control and accurate ingredient measurements, ensuring consistency in meal preparation. By incorporating these kitchen gadgets into their culinary arsenal, individuals can navigate the challenges of cooking post-colostomy surgery with ease and confidence.

CHAPTER 9

DINING OUT AND SOCIALIZING WITH CONFIDENCE

When recovering from surgery, particularly one involving a colostomy, adapting to a new way of eating can be challenging. However, it's crucial not to let dietary restrictions hinder one's ability to enjoy dining out or socializing with friends and family. In this section, we will explore strategies for navigating menus with dietary restrictions, offer tips for eating out safely, and provide advice for hosting gatherings and parties while managing a colostomy recovery.

Navigating Menus with Dietary Restrictions

Navigating menus with dietary restrictions, especially in the context of colostomy recovery, requires a proactive approach and effective communication.

Firstly, it's essential to research restaurants in advance, looking for those with a variety of options and a willingness to accommodate special dietary needs.

Many restaurants now provide their menus online, making it easier to assess whether they offer suitable choices for individuals with colostomies.

When reviewing menus, focus on dishes that are easily digestible, low in fiber, and unlikely to cause discomfort or digestive issues. Grilled or baked proteins such as chicken, fish, or tofu are generally safe options, as are well-cooked vegetables without skins or seeds. Additionally, inquire about the preparation methods used by the restaurant to ensure they align with your dietary requirements.

If you're unsure about a particular dish or ingredient, don't hesitate to ask your server for clarification. Most restaurants are accustomed to catering to various dietary needs and will be happy to accommodate reasonable requests.

Moreover, consider speaking directly with the chef or kitchen staff to discuss your needs in more detail and ensure a safe and enjoyable dining experience.

Tips for Eating Out Safely

Eating out safely while recovering from colostomy surgery requires mindfulness and preparation. Firstly, it's essential to plan by researching restaurants and reviewing their menus to identify suitable options. Choose establishments known for their flexibility and willingness to accommodate dietary restrictions.

When dining out, communicate your dietary needs clearly and assertively to your server. Be specific about any ingredients or cooking methods to avoid, such as high-fiber foods, seeds, or spicy seasonings that may irritate the digestive system.

Don't hesitate to ask for modifications to dishes to better suit your needs, such as requesting sauces or dressings on the side or substituting certain ingredients.

Additionally, be mindful of portion sizes and pace yourself while eating. Overeating or consuming rich, heavy foods can put unnecessary strain on the digestive system, potentially leading to discomfort or complications. Consider ordering smaller portions or sharing dishes with dining companions to avoid overwhelming your system.

Lastly, be prepared with any necessary supplies or medications, such as digestive enzymes or anti-diarrheal medications, in case of unexpected issues while dining out. By taking a proactive approach and advocating for your dietary needs, you can enjoy meals outside the home with confidence and peace of mind.

Hosting Gatherings and Parties

Hosting gatherings and parties can be enjoyable and rewarding, even when managing a colostomy recovery. However, it requires careful planning and consideration to ensure that all guests, including those with dietary restrictions, feel comfortable and included.

Firstly, when planning the menu for your event, consider offering a variety of options to accommodate different dietary needs and preferences. Include plenty of fresh fruits and vegetables, lean proteins, and whole grains, while avoiding foods that may be problematic for individuals with colostomies, such as high-fiber or spicy dishes.

Communicate with your guests in advance to inquire about any dietary restrictions or preferences they may have. This allows you to tailor the menu accordingly and ensure that everyone has something safe and enjoyable to eat. Consider labeling dishes with common allergens or dietary information to help guests make informed choices.

When hosting a gathering, provide a comfortable and private space for guests who may need to attend to their ostomy appliances or take medications. Ensure that restroom facilities are easily accessible and well-stocked with any necessary supplies.

Additionally, be mindful of alcohol consumption, as it can affect digestion and exacerbate symptoms for some individuals. Offer plenty of non-alcoholic beverage options, such as water, herbal teas, or mocktails, to ensure that all guests feel included and comfortable.

Overall, hosting gatherings and parties while managing a colostomy recovery requires sensitivity, flexibility, and attention to detail. By planning, communicating effectively, and prioritizing the needs of all guests, you can create a welcoming and inclusive environment where everyone can relax and enjoy themselves.

CHAPTER 10
EMOTIONAL WELL-BEING AND RECOVERY

The journey of recovery following a colostomy surgery entails not only physical adjustments but also emotional resilience. Coping with emotional challenges is an integral aspect of the recovery process. Patients often grapple with feelings of loss, anxiety, and uncertainty as they adapt to the changes brought about by the surgery. Therefore, establishing effective coping strategies and nurturing emotional well-being are paramount to achieving holistic recovery.

Coping Strategies for Emotional Challenges

Navigating the emotional landscape post-colostomy surgery requires employing coping strategies tailored to individual needs and circumstances. Firstly, fostering self-compassion is essential.

Patients must acknowledge their feelings without judgment and treat themselves with kindness and understanding. Embracing a positive mindset can significantly impact one's emotional well-being. Engaging in mindfulness practices such as meditation and deep breathing exercises can help alleviate stress and promote a sense of calm amidst turbulent emotions.

Furthermore, maintaining open communication with healthcare providers, friends, and family members can provide invaluable support. Sharing concerns and seeking guidance from medical professionals can alleviate anxieties and facilitate a smoother transition to life with a colostomy. Additionally, connecting with support groups or online communities comprised of individuals who have undergone similar experiences can offer a sense of solidarity and belonging.

Practicing resilience is another vital coping strategy. Recognizing setbacks as temporary challenges rather than insurmountable obstacles can empower patients to persevere through difficult times. Setting realistic goals and celebrating small victories along the way can foster a sense of accomplishment and boost morale. Moreover, engaging in activities that bring joy and fulfillment, such as hobbies or creative outlets, can serve as effective distractions from negative emotions.

Lastly, seeking professional counseling or therapy can be beneficial for individuals struggling to cope with emotional challenges post-surgery. Therapists can provide strategies for managing stress, processing feelings of grief or loss, and fostering resilience. Additionally, cognitive-behavioral therapy techniques can help patients reframe negative thoughts and develop coping mechanisms for dealing with anxiety or depression.

Mindful Eating Practices

Mindful eating entails fostering mindfulness and concentration during meals, which can build a healthy connection with food and improve the body's healing process post-colostomy surgery. Adopting mindful eating techniques can help patients reconnect with their bodies, promote digestion, and maximize nutritional absorption.

One important part of mindful eating is paying attention to hunger and satiety indicators. Eating deliberately and Savoring each meal encourages individuals to identify sensations of fullness and prevent overeating, which can lead to pain or digestive disorders. Additionally, expressing thankfulness for the sustenance supplied by food may build a greater appreciation for meals and promote a positive attitude towards eating.

Furthermore, being careful of dietary choices is vital for aiding post-surgery healing. Opting for nutrient-dense, whole meals such as fruits, vegetables, lean meats, and whole grains can give critical vitamins, minerals, and fiber necessary for healing and general well-being. Incorporating a range of colors and textures into meals not only makes dining more fun but also assures a wide assortment of nutrients.

Moreover, adopting careful portion management can help reduce digestive pain and maintain a healthy weight post-surgery. Using smaller plates, and serving sizes, and being conscious of portion sizes helps minimize overindulgence and encourage healthier digestion. Additionally, responding to the body's hunger and fullness cues helps regulate portion sizes and reduce needless calorie consumption.

Incorporating mindfulness into meal preparation and cooking may also enhance the dining experience. Engaging all the senses when cooking, such as examining colors, textures, and scents, may heighten appreciation for food and boost enjoyment. Additionally, including loved ones in meal preparation may build a sense of connection and satisfaction surrounding eating.

Building a Support Network

Building a strong support network is vital for those having colostomy surgery and subsequent rehabilitation. A comprehensive support system may give emotional encouragement, practical aid, and essential resources to negotiate the obstacles of post-surgery living.

Family members and friends play a significant role in offering emotional support and encouragement during the rehabilitation process. For patients getting used to living with a colostomy, their confidence and presence can ease fears and provide them comfort. Furthermore, family members may help with everyday responsibilities like food preparation, housework, and transportation to doctor's appointments, relieving patients of some of the stress while they concentrate on getting better.

A patient's support network includes important healthcare providers in addition to personal relationships.

To meet the particular requirements of people with colostomies, physicians, nurses, dietitians, and other healthcare providers can provide direction, instruction, and specialized treatment. Maintaining open lines of contact with medical professionals guarantees that patients get all the assistance they need as they recuperate.

Joining online forums or support groups made up of others who have gone through similar things may also foster understanding and a sense of solidarity. By establishing connections with other individuals who have had colostomy surgery, patients can seek support from peers who can relate to their experience, share ideas, and offer advice. These groups provide a secure environment where people may share their worries, commemorate achievements, and get support from those who are aware of the difficulties associated with having a colostomy.

Furthermore, those who are having a hard time managing the emotional effects of colostomy surgery may find it helpful to seek out professional counseling or therapy. Therapists can offer a safe space where patients can explore their emotions, create coping mechanisms, and deal with any psychological issues that may have resulted from the procedure. Counseling sessions may also assist patients in resolving problems with intimacy, body image, and self-esteem, promoting acceptance and empowerment.

creating a network of friends, family, medical experts, and peers is crucial for fostering mental wellness and expediting the healing process after colostomy surgery. Through cultivating relationships, pursuing assistance, and engaging in self-maintenance, people may effectively confront the difficulties of life after surgery with fortitude and hope.

CONCLUSION

A multidisciplinary strategy combining culinary innovation, mental fortitude, and nutritional knowledge is necessary to navigate the path of colostomy rehabilitation. Every detail of this extensive guide, from the fundamentals of balanced nutrition explained in Chapter 1 to the decadent yet health-conscious desserts in Chapter 6, has been painstakingly designed to assist you on your path to recovery.

You give yourself the best chance of a good recovery by being aware of the subtleties of colostomy recovery and following the dietary recommendations. The therapeutic recipes in Chapters 2 through 4 provide a wide range of alternatives to suit your palate and dietary requirements, whether you're in the mood for nutrient-dense oats for breakfast or hearty one-pot meals for lunch.

Apart from providing filling meals, Chapter 5 emphasizes the need for mindful snacking and provides inventive suggestions for healthful sides so that every bite enhances your overall well-being. In the meantime, Chapter 7 offers a delightful selection of drinks to sustain your energy and hydration levels throughout the day.

Recognizing the entire aspect of rehabilitation, this book goes beyond diet to include cooking methods, eating-out tactics, and activities for mental well-being. Every aspect of your journey is welcomed and encouraged, from flavor-enhancing ingredients to convenient cooking tools, from establishing mindful eating habits to confidently navigating social settings.

As you set out on your journey to sustained well-being, keep in mind that emotional as well as physical healing occurs. In Chapter 10, the significance of developing a strong support system, practicing mindful eating, and developing coping mechanisms is emphasized as ways to deal with potential emotional obstacles.

This all-inclusive handbook essentially acts as a lighthouse of direction and encouragement, pointing the way toward the best possible recovery after surgery and long-term well-being. I hope it gives you the courage, fortitude, and steadfast dedication to your well-being to face your path head-on.